Metabolic Confusion Diet

A Beginner's 5-Step Plan and Overview on Its Use Cases, Including Weight Loss

copyright © 2024 Stephanie Hinderock

All rights reserved No part of this book may be reproduced, or stored in a retrieval system, or transmitted in any form or by any means, electronic, mechanical, photocopying, recording, or otherwise, without express written permission of the publisher.

Disclaimer

By reading this disclaimer, you are accepting the terms of the disclaimer in full. If you disagree with this disclaimer, please do not read the guide.

All of the content within this guide is provided for informational and educational purposes only, and should not be accepted as independent medical or other professional advice. The author is not a doctor, physician, nurse, mental health provider, or registered nutritionist/dietician. Therefore, using and reading this guide does not establish any form of a physician-patient relationship.

Always consult with a physician or another qualified health provider with any issues or questions you might have regarding any sort of medical condition. Do not ever disregard any qualified professional medical advice or delay seeking that advice because of anything you have read in this guide. The information in this guide is not intended to be any sort of medical advice and should not be used in lieu of any medical advice by a licensed and qualified medical professional.

The information in this guide has been compiled from a variety of known sources. However, the author cannot attest to or guarantee the accuracy of each source and thus should not be held liable for any errors or omissions.

You acknowledge that the publisher of this guide will not be held liable for any loss or damage of any kind incurred as a result of this guide or the reliance on any information provided within this guide. You acknowledge and agree that you assume all risk and responsibility for any action you undertake in response to the information in this guide.

Using this guide does not guarantee any particular result (e.g., weight loss or a cure). By reading this guide, you acknowledge that there are no guarantees to any specific outcome or results you can expect.

All product names, diet plans, or names used in this guide are for identification purposes only and are the property of their respective owners. The use of these names does not imply endorsement. All other trademarks cited herein are the property of their respective owners.

Where applicable, this guide is not intended to be a substitute for the original work of this diet plan and is, at most, a supplement to the original work for this diet plan and never a direct substitute. This guide is a personal expression of the facts of that diet plan.

Where applicable, persons shown in the cover images are stock photography models and the publisher has obtained the rights to use the images through license agreements with third-party stock image companies.

Table of Contents

Introduction	7
Understanding Metabolic Confusion Diet	9
Understanding Metabolism	9
Metabolic Confusion Diet	10
Principles of Metabolic Confusion Diet	11
Benefits of Metabolic Confusion Diet	15
Use Cases of Metabolic Confusion Diet	18
Obesity	18
Type 2 Diabetes	18
Heart Disease	19
High Blood Pressure	19
High Cholesterol	20
Polycystic Ovary Syndrome (PCOS)	20
Pros and Cons	22
Advantages of Metabolic Confusion Diet	22
Disadvantages of Metabolic Confusion Diet	23
What Women Should Be Aware of Regarding this Diet?	26
Who Should Try the Metabolic Confusion Diet	29
Who Shouldn't Try the Metabolic Confusion Diet	30
Step-by-Step Guide on How to Get Started With Metabolic Confusion Diet for Women	32
Step 1: Consult a healthcare professional	32
Step 2: Calculate your daily calorie needs	33
Step 3: Determine Macronutrient Ratio Goals	34
Step 4: Create a Meal Plan	34
Step 5: Track your progress	35
Foods to Eat	36
Foods to Avoid	40
Phases of Metabolic Confusion Diet	43

Phase 1: High-Calorie Day (Boost Metabolism)	43
Phase 2: Low-Calorie Day (Promote Weight Loss)	44
Phase 3: Medium-Calorie Day (Maintain Metabolic Flexibility)	45
Exercise Routines to Boost the Metabolic Confusion Diet	45
Addressing common challenges and potential pitfalls that women may encounter while following the metabolic confusion diet:	49
Sample Recipes and Meal Plan	**52**
Mashed Sweet Potato topped with Sautéed Spinach, Mushrooms, and a Fried Egg	53
Quinoa Bowl with Black Beans, Roasted Vegetables, and Grilled Salmon	55
Baked Salmon with Roasted Asparagus and Quinoa	57
Apple Slices with Almond Butter	59
Protein Shake with Banana and Peanut Butter	60
Roasted Chickpeas	61
Overnight Oats with Blueberries, Almond Milk, and Protein Powder	62
Green Salad with Grilled Chicken, Feta Cheese, and Light Vinaigrette	63
Ingredients:	63
Carrot Sticks with Hummus	64
Baked Tilapia with Steamed Broccoli, Cauliflower, and Brown Rice	66
Sample Meal Plan	67
Conclusion	**71**
FAQ	**74**
References and Helpful Links	**76**

Introduction

Are you feeling frustrated and discouraged by the continuous cycle of fad diets that promise quick results but ultimately fail to deliver? If you're prepared for a genuinely transformative weight loss experience that goes beyond mere hollow promises, then the innovative Metabolic Confusion Diet is the answer you've been earnestly seeking.

By harnessing the power of your body's metabolism, the Metabolic Confusion Diet challenges conventional dieting methods and keeps your body guessing, preventing frustrating plateaus and maximizing your fat-burning potential. It's time to break free from the never-ending cycle of restrictive diets that leave you feeling deprived and unsatisfied. With the Metabolic Confusion Diet, you can finally discover a new and effective approach that truly works.

Imagine a diet where you can enjoy a wide variety of delicious and nutritious foods, never feeling deprived or restricted. Picture consistently witnessing the numbers on the scale drop week after week, as your body effortlessly sheds unwanted pounds. With the Metabolic Confusion Diet, this dream can become your reality.

Achieve accelerated fat loss, boosted energy, sharper mental focus, and improved metabolic flexibility with this groundbreaking approach. This comprehensive guide will help you understand the science behind the Metabolic Confusion Diet and seamlessly integrate it into your lifestyle for optimal and lasting results.

In this Guide, we will talk about the following;

- Understanding Metabolic Confusion Diet
- Use Cases
- Principles and Benefits of Metabolic Confusion Diet
- Pros and Cons
- What Women Should Be Aware of Regarding This Diet
- Who Should and Shouldn't Try the Metabolic Confusion Diet?
- Step Guide on How to Get Started With Metabolic Confusion Diet for Women
- Foods to Eat and To Avoid
- Phases of Metabolic Confusion Diet
- Sample Recipes and Meal Plan

Keep reading this comprehensive guide to learn more about the Metabolic Confusion Diet and how you can implement it into your lifestyle for optimal results.

Understanding Metabolic Confusion Diet

Understanding Metabolism

Metabolism is a complex process that your body uses to convert the food you eat into energy. This energy is then used for everything from moving around to thinking to growing. Your metabolism comprises two key parts:

Anabolism

Anabolism is one of the two key parts of metabolism, alongside catabolism. It is the metabolic process that requires energy to create cells or repair and maintain tissues. This process involves the synthesis of complex molecules from simpler ones, such as protein synthesis from amino acids.

Anabolism is essential for the growth, development, and maintenance of bodily structures, such as bones, muscles, and organs. Additionally, anabolic reactions require enzymes to catalyze the chemical reactions involved, and they are often regulated by hormones such as insulin and growth hormone.

Overall, anabolism plays a critical role in maintaining the proper functioning of the body's tissues and processes.

Catabolism

Anabolism builds the body's tissues and organs, while catabolism breaks down food into energy. This process occurs in all cells, breaking down complex molecules like carbohydrates, fats, and proteins into simpler ones for energy production.

The released energy fuels cellular processes, including muscle contraction and body temperature regulation. Catabolism results in carbon dioxide, water, and energy, vital for the body's needs. Metabolic rate varies based on age, gender, physical activity, and genetics.

Metabolic Confusion Diet

A metabolic confusion diet, also known as calorie cycling, is a dietary approach based on the idea of keeping your metabolism active and preventing it from getting used to a certain level of calorie intake. The theory suggests that by regularly changing your calorie intake, your body is kept guessing, and this prevents your metabolism from slowing down, which often happens with consistent low-calorie diets.

A typical metabolic confusion diet might involve alternating between high-calorie and low-calorie days. For example, you may follow a low-calorie diet for two days, followed by a high-calorie diet for the next two days, and so on. The exact ratio of high to low-calorie days can vary depending on individual goals and preferences.

However, it's important to note that while this approach may work for some, it may not be suitable for everyone, and more research is needed to fully understand its potential benefits and drawbacks. Always consult with a healthcare professional before starting any new diet regimen.

Principles of Metabolic Confusion Diet

The metabolic confusion diet is based on the following principles:

Calorie Cycling

The metabolic confusion diet is a unique approach that involves strategically alternating between high-calorie and low-calorie intake. On high-calorie days, women consume a slightly higher amount of calories, ensuring they have ample energy and essential nutrients to support their active lifestyle. Conversely, during low-calorie days, they significantly reduce their calorie intake, creating a slight calorie deficit.

This fluctuation in calorie intake keeps the metabolism on its toes, preventing it from becoming too adaptive to a specific calorie level. By continuously challenging the metabolism, the goal of this diet is to encourage fat burning, even during periods of rest. This approach not only aids in weight loss but also aims to maintain a healthy metabolic rate for overall well-being and sustained results.

Macronutrient Variation

In the metabolic confusion diet, women strategically adjust their macronutrient ratios, altering the proportions of carbohydrates, proteins, and fats consumed on different days. This deliberate variation in nutrient composition challenges the body to efficiently process and utilize a diverse range of nutrients, thereby potentially stimulating the metabolism and enhancing calorie-burning efficiency for effective weight loss.

Moreover, this approach not only aids in achieving weight loss goals but also promotes a well-rounded nutrient intake, ensuring overall health, vitality, and well-being. By incorporating this method into their dietary routine, women can embark on a holistic journey towards improved fitness and a balanced lifestyle.

Meal Planning and Preparation

To effectively implement the metabolic confusion diet, meticulous meal planning, period and preparation are key. Women can strategically strategize and curate their meals, ensuring they align with the desired calorie and macronutrient targets for each phase of the diet.

By carefully preparing meals in advance, individuals can enhance adherence to the prescribed calorie intake, making it easier to stay on track and achieve their goals. This attention to detail and proactive approach can contribute to long-term success and optimal results.

Regular Exercise

Incorporating regular exercise is a fundamental principle of the metabolic confusion diet for women. By engaging in a variety of physical activities, such as cardiovascular exercises, strength training, and other dynamic workouts, you can effectively boost your metabolism, burn calories, and support your overall weight-loss efforts.

Additionally, regular exercise not only helps with weight management but also improves cardiovascular health, increases muscle tone, and enhances overall well-being. So, by diversifying your exercise routine and staying consistent, you can maximize the benefits of the metabolic confusion diet and achieve your fitness goals with greater success.

Monitoring Progress

Women who are following the metabolic confusion diet should diligently monitor their progress to gain a comprehensive understanding of its effectiveness. It is recommended to track various metrics, including weight, body measurements, energy levels, and overall well-being.

By regularly monitoring these aspects, individuals can gain valuable insights into their body's response to the diet and make necessary adjustments for optimal results. This continuous monitoring and fine-tuning approach ensures that the diet is tailored to each individual's unique needs and goals, ultimately leading to better outcomes.

Long-Term Sustainability

The metabolic confusion diet for women places great emphasis on the significance of long-term sustainability and adherence to achieve optimal results. While this diet may yield initial weight loss, it recognizes the importance of maintaining a healthy lifestyle beyond the diet phase. It encourages women to adopt sustainable eating habits that are enjoyable and nourishing, ensuring that they can sustain their progress over time.

Additionally, incorporating regular exercise into their routine and making gradual, realistic changes will further support their journey towards lasting success in achieving their weight loss goals. By focusing on these holistic approaches, women can cultivate a positive relationship with food, exercise, and their overall well-being.

When followed properly, the metabolic confusion diet can be a safe and effective approach to weight loss for women. This comprehensive guide will cover everything you need to know to get started on this diet and maximize your success.

Benefits of Metabolic Confusion Diet

The Metabolic Confusion Diet for women offers numerous benefits, including;

Weight Loss

The metabolic confusion diet is particularly beneficial for women who want to lose weight. Its calorie cycling and macronutrient variation can help not only create a calorie deficit but also stimulate the metabolism, leading to increased fat burning. This is because the body can adapt to a consistent diet and begin to conserve energy, making it harder to lose weight.

However, with the metabolic confusion diet, the body is constantly challenged with variations in calorie intake and macronutrient ratios, which keeps the metabolism guessing and in turn, burns more calories.

Metabolic Boost

The metabolic confusion diet has been touted as an effective way to boost metabolism specifically for women. The alternating patterns of calorie intake and macronutrient ratios that the diet recommends keep the body guessing and working harder to process different foods. This can lead to an elevated metabolic rate, resulting in increased calorie burn and overall improved well-being.

Muscle Preservation

The metabolic confusion diet can also help women preserve their muscle mass during weight loss. Its emphasis on a balanced macronutrient intake and regular physical activity can ensure that the body is getting enough of each nutrient to maintain healthy muscles, while still burning fat. This combination helps to maximize the effects of the diet and ensures lasting weight loss results.

Reduced Plateau Effect

The metabolic confusion diet can also help to reduce the plateau effect that often occurs with weight loss. By alternating between calorie levels and macronutrient ratios, it keeps the body guessing and prevents it from becoming too adaptive—which can lead to a slowing down of metabolism and plateaus in weight loss progress.

Improved Insulin Sensitivity

Insulin sensitivity is an important factor for women looking to maintain a healthy weight. The metabolic confusion diet can help improve insulin sensitivity by promoting the consumption of whole foods, such as fruits and vegetables, which are rich in fiber and other beneficial nutrients that help regulate blood sugar levels. Additionally, its variable macronutrient ratios can also support better insulin response and healthier energy levels.

Incorporating the metabolic confusion diet into your lifestyle can offer numerous health benefits. However, there are a few things that women should be aware of when following this approach to weight loss.

Use Cases of Metabolic Confusion Diet

The following are some of the most common use cases for the metabolic confusion diet:

Obesity

Obesity is a widespread health issue with various complications. The Metabolic Confusion diet tackles obesity by keeping the metabolism active and burning calories more efficiently. This diet alternates between high and low-calorie days, confusing the metabolism, and promoting weight loss.

It promotes consistent metabolic activity, aiding weight reduction and preventing weight regain, a common problem with traditional diets. A promising approach for obesity, providing a sustainable and effective weight loss solution.

Type 2 Diabetes

Type 2 Diabetes is a chronic condition that affects blood sugar processing. The Metabolic Confusion diet may help manage blood sugar levels, reducing the risk or severity of this disease. By alternating high and low-calorie intake days, this diet maintains consistent blood sugar levels, preventing spikes and crashes that worsen diabetes symptoms.

Additionally, weight loss improves insulin sensitivity, further aiding in blood sugar control. The Metabolic Confusion diet offers an innovative approach to diabetes management, promoting healthier eating patterns and potentially mitigating this prevalent condition.

Heart Disease

Heart disease remains a leading cause of death worldwide. The Metabolic Confusion diet, by promoting weight loss and healthy eating habits, may indirectly contribute to heart health. Weight loss is often associated with lower blood pressure and cholesterol levels, two significant risk factors for heart disease.

Additionally, the varied nutrient intake from alternating high and low-calorie days can ensure a balanced diet, further supporting cardiovascular health. Therefore, this diet may offer an additional tool in the fight against heart disease.

High Blood Pressure

High blood pressure, or hypertension, is a significant risk factor for heart disease and stroke. Weight loss, which can be a result of the metabolic confusion diet, often leads to lower blood pressure. This diet's alternating calorie intake keeps the metabolism active, promoting weight loss and indirectly contributing to blood pressure management.

Also, healthier eating patterns encouraged by this diet could lead to a reduction in sodium intake, a known contributor to high blood pressure. Thus, this diet may aid in controlling hypertension.

High Cholesterol

High cholesterol is a silent threat that can lead to serious heart conditions. The Metabolic Confusion diet encourages the consumption of healthy fats, such as omega-3 fatty acids, and lean proteins, which can help manage cholesterol levels.

By reducing intake of saturated fats and replacing them with healthier options, this diet may decrease LDL (bad cholesterol) and increase HDL (good cholesterol). Furthermore, weight loss associated with this diet can also positively impact cholesterol levels, making this regimen potentially beneficial for individuals with high cholesterol.

Polycystic Ovary Syndrome (PCOS)

Polycystic Ovary Syndrome (PCOS) is a hormonal disorder common among women of reproductive age. Some studies suggest that changes in diet can help manage PCOS symptoms, and the metabolic confusion diet might be one such beneficial dietary change.

This diet which alternates between high and low-calorie days, could potentially aid in weight loss, improve insulin sensitivity, and balance hormone levels - all key factors in managing PCOS. In addition, the focus on lean proteins and healthy fats may also help regulate blood sugar levels, providing further benefits for individuals with PCOS.

Please note that while the metabolic confusion diet may help manage these conditions, it's not a guaranteed cure or treatment. Always consult with a healthcare professional before starting any new diet plan.

Pros and Cons

When considering the metabolic confusion diet, it is important to understand both its advantages and drawbacks. Here are some of the pros and cons of this approach to weight loss for women.

Advantages of Metabolic Confusion Diet

Variety of Nutrients

The metabolic confusion diet offers a variety of nutrients, which can provide numerous health benefits. Alternating between calorie levels and macronutrient ratios ensures that the body is getting enough of each necessary nutrient while also providing enough variety to keep the metabolism stimulated. This helps support overall health and well-being in addition to weight loss.

Avoids Metabolic Adaptation

The metabolic confusion diet avoids the metabolic adaptation that often occurs with other diets, meaning it can be used for long-term weight loss. Varying calorie levels and macronutrient ratios, keep the body guessing and prevent it from becoming too adaptive - which can lead to a slowing down of metabolism and plateaus in weight loss progress.

No Severe Calorie Restriction

In contrast to many other diets, the metabolic confusion diet does not involve severe calorie restriction or elimination of certain foods. Instead, it encourages individuals to eat a balanced diet while varying their macronutrient intake and calories to achieve their desired weight loss goals.

Sustainability

The metabolic confusion diet is a sustainable approach to weight loss. Its emphasis on long-term habits and gradual lifestyle changes ensures that individuals can maintain their weight when the diet phase is complete, without reverting to old behaviors.

Remember, while these are potential advantages, individual experiences may vary. Always consult with a healthcare professional before starting any new diet regimen.

Disadvantages of Metabolic Confusion Diet

While the Metabolic Confusion Diet offers various benefits, such as weight loss and increased metabolism, it is important to consider the potential disadvantages. These include:

Focus on Calories Over Nutrients

Women who follow the metabolic confusion diet may be at risk of nutrient deficiencies due to its focus on calorie intake. This may result in insufficient amounts of vitamins, minerals, and macronutrients, particularly on low-calorie days. As a result, their bodies may not receive the necessary fuel and building blocks for optimal health and functioning.

Nutrient deficiencies can have a wide range of adverse health effects. For example, a weakened immune function can make individuals more susceptible to infections and illnesses. Impaired cognitive function may affect memory, concentration, and overall mental performance.

Potential Health Risks

Women who choose to follow the metabolic confusion diet should be mindful of potential health risks associated with its emphasis on calorie cycling. If calorie intake is consistently too low or not properly balanced, it can result in nutrient deficiencies and other negative effects on overall health.

Moreover, the frequent fluctuations in macronutrient composition may contribute to digestive problems, including bloating and indigestion. It is important for individuals considering this diet to be aware of these factors and to consult with a healthcare professional before making any significant dietary changes.

Difficulty Sticking to Schedule

Maintaining a consistent diet schedule can be quite challenging, especially for women with busy lifestyles, when following the metabolic confusion diet. This unique approach involves alternating calorie levels and macronutrient ratios, demanding strict adherence to maximize results.

However, due to the complexity of the diet, it can be difficult to sustain over an extended periodhurt. Therefore, it requires not only dedication but also careful planning and organization to ensure long-term success.

Not Holistic

The metabolic confusion diet, although popular, is not considered a holistic approach to weight loss. While it does focus on calorie restriction and macronutrient cycling, it fails to address other crucial factors that play a significant role in overall health and successful long-term weight management.

Factors like stress levels, sleep quality, and lifestyle habits are equally important and should not be overlooked. Balancing these elements is key to achieving and maintaining optimal health and sustainable weight loss goals.

Despite these potential disadvantages, when done healthily and responsibly, the metabolic confusion diet for women can be an effective approach to weight loss.

What Women Should Be Aware of Regarding this Diet?

When following the metabolic confusion diet, it's important to be aware of the potential risks and side effects. This includes:

Hormonal Imbalances

In addition to potential disruptions in menstrual cycles and fertility problems, a diet that lacks consistency and stability may also lead to hormonal imbalances in women. This is because fluctuating caloric intake can make it difficult for the body to maintain adequate levels of hormones such as estrogen, progesterone, and testosterone.

Hormonal imbalances not only affect reproductive health but can also affect mood, energy levels, and stress responses. Women need to be mindful of their caloric intake and nutrient intake to ensure hormonal balance and overall well-being.

Risk of Nutrient Deficiency

Women who follow a metabolic confusion diet should be cautious as they may not consume enough nutrients, leading to deficiencies of vital minerals such as iron and calcium. Iron is crucial for red blood cell formation and transporting oxygen in the body, while calcium is vital for bone formation and healthy nerve and muscle function.

Deficiencies of these nutrients can lead to anemia, osteoporosis, and muscle cramps, among other issues. It is recommended that women on such a diet should monitor their nutrient intake and consider taking supplements if necessary.

Potential for Disordered Eating

Women with a history of eating disorders or body image struggles may be particularly prone to disordered eating patterns while following a metabolic confusion diet. Calorie counting and cycling may trigger obsessions with food and weight, ultimately leading to negative mental and physical health consequences.

Women with a history of disordered eating need to work with a healthcare professional to develop a safe and healthy eating plan that doesn't trigger their old patterns.

Increased Stress Levels

One of the major side effects of this diet is an increase in stress levels. Women are forced to constantly monitor their caloric intake, which can cause mental and emotional exhaustion. Chronic stress, a common result of this diet, has been linked to various health problems, including an increased risk of heart disease and depression.

It is important to note that this diet may not be suitable for everyone and that a balanced and sustainable approach should always be taken when considering weight loss.

Impact on Bone Health

If not properly managed, these diets can have negative impacts on bone health, especially for women who are already at a higher risk of osteoporosis. Inadequate calcium intake is a common side effect of low-calorie days that are often a part of metabolic confusion diets. Calcium is essential for the maintenance of strong bones, and a deficiency can lead to a higher risk of fractures and osteoporosis.

Women are particularly vulnerable to this, and anyone following a metabolic confusion diet must ensure that they consume enough calcium through their food or supplements. Calcium-rich foods include dairy products, leafy greens, and fortified foods, but it is advisable to consult with a healthcare professional to determine the appropriate level of calcium intake and the need for supplements.

Effects on Physical Performance

On low-calorie days, the metabolic confusion diet can significantly affect the physical performance of women. The combination of reduced energy availability and increased energy demands from physical activity poses a challenge for active women or athletes. Inadequate energy intake can lead to fatigue, weakness, and decreased endurance, limiting performance.

Additionally, inefficient fueling may cause muscle loss, further impacting strength and power. Women on the metabolic confusion diet should be cautious, consuming enough calories to meet their energy demands for better performance. Remember, individual experiences may vary, and it's essential to consult a healthcare professional before starting any new diet.

Who Should Try the Metabolic Confusion Diet

People Seeking Weight Loss

For individuals pursuing weight loss, the Metabolic Confusion Diet could prove useful. The strategy of varying between days of high and low-calorie consumption is considered to stimulate your metabolism, thereby enhancing its ability to burn calories effectively.

Fitness Enthusiasts

Those who regularly participate in strenuous workouts could find value in this diet. High-calorie days provide ample energy for their exercise routines, while low-calorie days may contribute to rest, recuperation, and shedding of fat.

Individuals Who Appreciate Diversity: This dietary approach permits an extensive assortment of foods and doesn't explicitly prohibit specific food categories. If you take pleasure in sampling various dishes and aren't fond of limiting diets, this could be an ideal choice for you.

Who Shouldn't Try the Metabolic Confusion Diet

Individuals Struggling with Eating Disorders

The diet's emphasis on monitoring and alternating caloric intake might inadvertently provoke unhealthy eating habits. Those who have previously battled with eating disorders should steer clear of this diet.

People with Specific Health Issues

Those who have medical conditions like diabetes, cardiovascular disease, or any health concern necessitating a regulated diet should abstain from trying the metabolic confusion diet unless under the guidance of a healthcare professional.

Women in the stages of Pregnancy or Lactation

These individuals have distinct nutritional demands that may not be fulfilled by the inconsistent calorie intake associated with this diet.

People Seeking Long-Term Sustainable Diet

Certain health professionals suggest that the metabolic confusion diet may not be a viable strategy for maintaining weight over an extended period. They assert that continually tracking and modifying calorie consumption can be mentally and emotionally draining, potentially making it unsustainable in the long run.

Remember, before starting any new diet plan, it's important to consult with a healthcare professional or registered dietitian. They can provide guidance based on your individual health needs and goals.

Step-by-Step Guide on How to Get Started With Metabolic Confusion Diet for Women

Incorporating the metabolic confusion diet into your lifestyle doesn't have to be difficult. Here is a step-by-step guide on how to get started with this diet plan for women;

Step 1: Consult a healthcare professional

Before starting any new diet plan, it's important to consult with a healthcare professional. They can provide personalized guidance based on your specific needs and health conditions. By actively seeking their advice, you can ensure that the diet plan you choose aligns with your goals and is safe for your overall well-being.

A healthcare professional will assess your medical history, current health status, and any underlying conditions that may impact your dietary choices. They have the knowledge and expertise to evaluate the risks and benefits of different diet plans, helping you make informed decisions.

They can also help you set realistic expectations and goals for your diet plan, offering valuable insights into proper nutrition, portion control, and balanced eating. This ensures that you meet your nutritional needs while working towards your desired outcomes.

Furthermore, consulting with a healthcare professional can help identify potential interactions between the diet plan and medications or supplements you may be taking. They can guide you in making necessary adjustments for optimal health and safety.

Remember, everyone's body is unique. By consulting with a healthcare professional, you prioritize your health and well-being, receiving personalized advice tailored to your needs.

Step 2: Calculate your daily calorie needs

The metabolic confusion diet is a unique approach that involves consuming varying amounts of calories on different days. To ensure you meet your daily calorie requirements, accurately calculate them by inputting your age, gender, weight, height, activity level, and goals into a reliable online calculator.

By calculating these values precisely, you can ensure optimal calorie intake while following the metabolic confusion diet. This personalized approach considers your specific needs, allowing you to tailor your calorie intake accordingly. Whether you want to lose weight, build muscle, or maintain your current physique, accurate calorie calculation is key to success with this diet.

Step 3: Determine Macronutrient Ratio Goals

To achieve optimal nutrition, determine your daily macronutrient ratio. This involves calculating the precise grams of protein, carbohydrates, and fats you should consume. Ensure a well-balanced and tailored intake to meet your specific needs. For muscle growth, increase protein and carbohydrate intake.

Options to calculate needs include online calculators or following a meal plan for the metabolic confusion diet. Optimizing macronutrient intake fuels your body and maximizes progress toward health and fitness goals. Whether weight loss, muscle gain, or overall well-being, macronutrient ratios are key to success.

Step 4: Create a Meal Plan

Once you've calculated your daily calorie and macronutrient needs, create a personalized meal plan with a variety of nutritious foods. Include fruits, vegetables, lean proteins, healthy fats, and complex carbohydrates.

Ensure your meals are balanced and provide essential vitamins and minerals. Incorporate different food groups for a wide range of nutrients, such as leafy greens for vitamin K and iron, citrus fruits for vitamin C, and dairy or fortified plant-based milk for calcium.

Consult a healthcare professional or dietitian for supplements if needed. Consider a meal plan for the metabolic confusion diet to boost metabolism. Experiment with foods and recipes to find what works best for you.

Step 5: Track your progress

Tracking your progress is crucial for success with the metabolic confusion diet. By diligently recording meals, calories, and macronutrient ratios, you can monitor goals and make necessary adjustments. An online tracking app is an effective way to track progress conveniently.

With detailed information, gain insights into how foods impact health. Analyze data to make informed decisions and optimize results. Monitoring progress visually through the app helps identify patterns and make further adjustments as needed. Take control of the metabolic confusion diet and achieve desired outcomes.

Following these steps can help you get started on your metabolic confusion diet journey. With proper planning and guidance, you can take control of your health and well-being and reach your goals in no time.

Foods to Eat

In the metabolic confusion diet, it is important to focus on consuming nutrient-dense foods that support your health and weight loss goals. Here are some foods that you can include in your metabolic confusion diet:

Lean Proteins

When it comes to the metabolic confusion diet for women, incorporating foods that provide lean proteins is crucial. These options include chicken breast, turkey, fish, tofu, beans, and lentils. They are excellent sources of essential amino acids that aid muscle preservation and growth.

Consuming these proteins is especially important when following an exercise routine, as they assist in repairing and building muscle tissue. Lean proteins are also beneficial in regulating metabolism and promoting weight loss, making them a staple in any nutritious diet plan.

Whole Grains

For women following the metabolic confusion diet, quinoa, brown rice, oats, and whole wheat bread are essential foods to eat. These whole grains provide a wealth of fiber, vitamins, and minerals that keep the body feeling full and satisfied.

Quinoa, in particular, is a superfood that's high in protein, iron, and magnesium.

Brown rice and oats are packed with essential nutrients like calcium, potassium, and B vitamins that help regulate hormones and boost metabolism. Whole wheat bread is another great source of fiber and nutrients, perfect for maintaining a healthy diet and feeling energized throughout the day. By incorporating these whole grains into their daily meals, women can ensure that their bodies are getting the nutrients they need to thrive.

Fruits and Vegetables

As part of the metabolic confusion diet for women, it's important to incorporate a variety of fruits and vegetables into your meals. Not only do they provide necessary vitamins and minerals but they also contain antioxidants that help protect your body from damage caused by free radicals.

Aim for a colorful plate to ensure you're getting a wide range of nutrients from different fruits and vegetables. Some great options include leafy greens, berries, citrus fruits, sweet potatoes, and bell peppers. It's recommended to have at least five servings of fruits and vegetables daily, so make sure to incorporate them into your snacks and meals throughout the day.

Healthy Fats

When it comes to the metabolic confusion diet for women, one important aspect is including healthy fats in your meal plan. Avocados are a great source of monounsaturated fats, which can help reduce bad cholesterol levels and lower the risk of heart disease.

Nuts, such as almonds and walnuts, are rich in omega-3 fatty acids that support brain health and reduce inflammation. Seeds, like chia and flax, are also high in omega-3s and fiber, which can aid in digestion and weight management.

Olive oil is a great alternative to saturated fats and can help with inflammation, digestive issues, and even cognitive function. All of these healthy fat sources should be consumed in moderation as part of a balanced diet.

Low-fat dairy or Dairy Alternatives

To effectively follow the metabolic confusion diet, women should focus on consuming low-fat dairy options such as Greek yogurt and cottage cheese, or opt for dairy alternatives like almond or soy milk.

These nutritious options provide an excellent source of both calcium and protein, which are essential for maintaining bone density and keeping muscles strong. Low-fat Greek yogurt, in particular, is an excellent choice for its high protein content and ability to keep you feeling full and satisfied for longer periods.

Additionally, dairy alternatives like almond milk and soy milk are great alternatives for those who are lactose intolerant or have a milk allergy. By incorporating these foods into your diet, you'll be able to maintain a healthy and balanced diet while simultaneously adhering to the metabolic confusion diet.

Hydrating Beverages

Hydrating beverages are crucial for anyone on a metabolic confusion diet aimed at promoting weight loss. In addition to plain water, herbal teas, and flavored water can provide some variety. However, it's essential to avoid sugary drinks that can derail your efforts.

The recommended daily intake for women is around 2.7 liters of fluids, and drinking water before meals helps to prevent overeating. Caffeine-free herbal teas, such as chamomile, ginger, mint, and dandelion root, can also promote digestion and reduce inflammation.

Finally, consider adding natural flavorings to your water, such as slices of cucumber, lemon, and mint, or even infusing it with berries or herbs for a refreshing and vitamin-rich drink.

Remember, portion control and balance are key in the metabolic confusion diet. Consult with a healthcare professional or registered dietitian for personalized guidance and recommendations based on your specific needs.

Foods to Avoid

In the metabolic confusion diet, there isn't a specific list of foods to avoid. The focus is primarily on calorie cycling and varying macronutrient ratios rather than specific food restrictions. However, it is generally recommended to limit or avoid foods that are high in added sugars, refined carbohydrates, and unhealthy fats. These may include:

Sugary Snacks and Beverages

Foods like candy, cookies, cakes, sodas, and sugary juices should be limited in consumption. These items are not only high in added sugars but also provide empty calories, which means they contribute to weight gain without offering any significant nutritional value.

By reducing the intake of these items, individuals can make healthier choices and prioritize nutrient-dense foods that support overall well-being.

Processed Foods

To maintain a healthy diet, it is advisable to steer clear of highly processed foods such as packaged snacks, frozen meals, and fast food. These types of foods often contain excessive amounts of unhealthy fats, high levels of sodium, and a variety of preservatives that can be detrimental to our well-being. By opting for fresh and natural alternatives, we can prioritize our health and make informed choices about what we consume.

Refined Grains

To promote a healthy diet, it is recommended to minimize the consumption of refined grains, such as white bread, white rice, and pasta. These types of grains undergo a process that strips them of fiber and essential nutrients, which are crucial for maintaining a balanced and nutritious diet.

By opting for whole grains instead, such as whole wheat bread, brown rice, and whole wheat pasta, you can ensure a higher intake of fiber and nutrients, contributing to your overall well-being.

Fried and High-Fat Foods

To promote a healthier lifestyle, it is advisable to limit the consumption of fried foods and those high in unhealthy fats. This includes avoiding deep-fried snacks, greasy fast-food items, and fatty cuts of meat, which can contribute to various health issues when consumed in excess. By making conscious choices and opting for alternative cooking methods, you can take a step towards improving your overall well-being.

Sweetened Condiments and Sauces

When selecting condiments and sauces, it's important to be mindful of their ingredients. Many commercially available options contain added sugars and unhealthy fats, which can hurt your health. Instead, consider opting for healthier alternatives or even making your own using natural, wholesome ingredients. By doing so, you can have better control over what you're consuming and make choices that support your overall well-being.

Remember, while these foods may be best to avoid or limit, it's also important to focus on consuming a variety of nutrient-dense foods that support your overall health and well-being. As always, individual needs and preferences may vary, so consult with a healthcare professional or registered dietitian for personalized guidance based on your specific goals and health conditions.

Phases of Metabolic Confusion Diet

The metabolic confusion diet typically involves cycling between different phases, each with a specific purpose. Here's a breakdown of the different phases of the metabolic confusion diet:

Phase 1: High-Calorie Day (Boost Metabolism)

Phase 1 of the metabolic confusion diet is the high-calorie day, which serves the purpose of boosting your metabolism. This phase involves consuming a higher calorie intake compared to the other phases of the diet. The rationale behind this is to prevent your body from adapting and slowing down its metabolic rate in response to lower calorie levels.

By having a high-calorie day, you give your metabolism a temporary boost, which can help prevent it from plateauing and becoming less efficient at burning calories. This temporary increase in calorie intake can also provide a psychological break from the lower-calorie days, making it easier to adhere to the overall diet plan.

Phase 2: Low-Calorie Day (Promote Weight Loss)

Phase 2 of the metabolic confusion diet is the low-calorie day, which is designed to promote weight loss. During this phase, you consume a reduced calorie intake compared to a high-calorie day. The purpose of the low-calorie day is to create a calorie deficit, where your body burns more calories than it takes in, leading to weight loss.

By consuming fewer calories, your body is encouraged to utilize stored fat as an energy source, leading to fat loss over time. This calorie deficit helps shift your body into a state where it is primarily relying on its fat stores for fuel, contributing to overall weight loss.

It's important to note that while the low-calorie day focuses on reducing calorie intake, it is still essential to prioritize nutrient-dense foods to ensure you are meeting your nutritional needs. Including a variety of fruits, vegetables, lean proteins, whole grains, and healthy fats can help provide essential vitamins, minerals, and other nutrients despite the lower calorie intake.

Phase 3: Medium-Calorie Day (Maintain Metabolic Flexibility)

Phase 3 of the metabolic confusion diet is the medium-calorie day, which serves the purpose of maintaining metabolic flexibility. This phase involves consuming a moderate calorie intake that falls between the higher and lower calorie days of the diet. The goal is to strike a balance between the high and low-calorie days, preventing your metabolism from adapting and becoming less efficient.

By incorporating medium-calorie days into the diet plan, you promote metabolic flexibility. This means that your body can efficiently switch between using different fuel sources, such as carbohydrates and fats, for energy. Maintaining metabolic flexibility can help prevent plateaus in weight loss and keep your metabolism functioning optimally.

The medium-calorie day still emphasizes the importance of nutrient-dense foods to support overall health and well-being. Including a variety of whole grains, lean proteins, fruits, vegetables, and healthy fats can help ensure that you meet your nutritional needs despite the moderate calorie intake.

Exercise Routines to Boost the Metabolic Confusion Diet

Cardiovascular Exercises

High-Intensity Interval Training (HIIT)

The Exercise Routine to Boost the Metabolic Confusion Diet involves a series of high-intensity exercises that alternate between periods of intense activity and recovery. This style of workout has been proven effective in boosting metabolism, helping women to burn fat and build lean muscle.

By forcing the body to constantly adapt to new levels of intensity, HIIT keeps the metabolism active and engaged, allowing for greater calorie burn both during and after the workout. Regularly practicing this type of exercise can help women achieve their weight loss and fitness goals more quickly and efficiently than traditional cardio or weight training routines.

Running or Jogging

Regular running or jogging sessions can greatly enhance the metabolic confusion diet for women, leading to better cardiovascular fitness. These exercises help increase oxygen consumption, calorie burning, and overall energy expenditure, promoting weight loss and improved health.

Running and jogging also release endorphins, reducing stress and helping to maintain mental health. Incorporating such exercises in the metabolic confusion diet can bring about optimal results and long-term benefits.

Cycling

Incorporating cycling into an exercise routine is a great way for women following the metabolic confusion diet to optimize their workouts. This low-impact exercise strengthens the heart and lungs, burns fat, promotes muscle growth, and improves overall fitness.

Additionally, cycling can be customized to fit various fitness levels and goals, as it can be done indoors or outdoors and at different intensities. It is a time-efficient exercise that can be done alone or with a group, making cycling a versatile and effective addition to any metabolic confusion diet plan.

Strength Training

Weightlifting

To boost the Metabolic Confusion Diet, women can incorporate weightlifting exercises using weights or resistance bands. This helps build muscle and increases metabolism, resulting in faster calorie burning. It also improves bone density and reduces the risk of osteoporosis. Incorporating weightlifting into your routine can have positive impacts on mental health by boosting self-esteem.

It can be done at home or in a gym, and different exercises can target specific muscle groups. It is crucial to use proper form and gradually increase weight to prevent injuries. Weightlifting coupled with a nutritional diet can create a sustainable healthy lifestyle.

Bodyweight Exercises

This exercise routine is perfect to boost the metabolic confusion diet for women. With push-ups, squats, lunges, and planks, you can use your body weight as resistance, allowing your muscles to strengthen and burn more calories.

These exercises also create metabolic confusion by engaging different muscle groups, increasing the rate of fat loss. Stick to this routine for great results!

Pilates or Yoga

Pilates and yoga are excellent exercise routines for women looking to boost their metabolic confusion diet. These practices not only improve strength, flexibility, and body awareness but also increase muscle mass and metabolic rate.

Pilates exercises specifically target the core muscles, leading to a stronger midsection and improved metabolism. Yoga, on the other hand, focuses on balancing the body's energy and reducing stress levels, which can also lead to an increased metabolic rate.

So, whether you choose to do Pilates or yoga, incorporating these practices into your daily routine can help boost your metabolism and support your weight loss goals.

Addressing common challenges and potential pitfalls that women may encounter while following the metabolic confusion diet:

Emotional Eating

Women may face challenges with emotional eating, a behavior triggered by stress, emotions, or social situations. This can lead to a cycle of unhealthy habits and negative impacts on physical and mental well-being. To break this cycle, it's important to develop alternative coping mechanisms.

One effective approach is practicing mindfulness, which involves being fully present and aware of your thoughts, feelings, and bodily sensations without judgment. Engaging in hobbies that bring joy and fulfillment can also provide a healthy distraction from emotional eating tendencies.

Additionally, seeking support from friends, family, or professionals who specialize in emotional health can be immensely helpful in overcoming this challenge and establishing a positive relationship with food and emotions.

Hormonal Fluctuations

Women may experience fluctuations in energy levels and appetite due to hormonal changes, such as during the menstrual cycle. These changes can create unique challenges when it comes to maintaining a balanced diet and managing overall well-being.

By actively listening to your body's cues and being mindful of these fluctuations, you can better understand your nutritional needs and make adjustments to your caloric intake accordingly. This self-awareness and responsiveness can go a long way in supporting your overall health and navigating these natural hormonal variations.

Unrealistic Expectations

It's crucial to set realistic expectations and prioritize overall health instead of solely focusing on weight loss. By celebrating non-scale victories, such as experiencing increased energy levels, improved mood, and enhanced fitness levels, you can truly appreciate the positive impact of your journey towards a healthier lifestyle. Embrace the little wins along the way and let them be the motivating force that propels you towards long-term success and well-being.

Lack of Planning

Planning meals and exercise in advance can be a game-changer when it comes to avoiding impulsive food choices and staying consistent with your diet and exercise routine. By taking the time to meal prep and schedule workouts ahead of time, you not only set yourself up for success but also create a sense of structure and control in your health and wellness journey.

This proactive approach allows you to make mindful choices, stick to your goals, and ultimately achieve the results you desire. So, why not give it a try and experience the benefits firsthand?

Remember, it's important to consult with a healthcare professional or a certified fitness trainer before starting any new exercise routine, especially if you have any underlying health conditions or concerns.

Sample Recipes and Meal Plan

Now that you have a better understanding of the metabolic confusion diet, here are some sample recipes and a meal plan to get you started. The meal plan provides an example of how to structure your meals based on the low, medium, and high-calorie days described in Chapter 3.

Mashed Sweet Potato topped with Sautéed Spinach, Mushrooms, and a Fried Egg

Ingredients:

- 2 medium sweet potatoes
- 1 tablespoon olive oil
- 2 cups spinach
- 1 cup sliced mushrooms
- 2 eggs
- Salt and pepper to taste

Instructions:

1. Preheat your oven to 400°F (200°C).
2. Scrub the sweet potatoes clean and prick them with a fork. Place them on a baking sheet and bake for about 45 minutes or until they are soft and can easily be mashed.
3. While the sweet potatoes are baking, heat olive oil in a pan over medium heat. Sauté the spinach and mushrooms until they are wilted and cooked through. Season with salt and pepper to taste.
4. In a separate pan, fry the eggs to your desired level of doneness.
5. Once the sweet potatoes are done baking, allow them to cool slightly. Peel off the skin and transfer the flesh to a mixing bowl. Mash the sweet potatoes with a fork until smooth.

6. To serve, divide the mashed sweet potatoes onto plates. Top with the sautéed spinach and mushrooms, and place a fried egg on top.
7. Season with additional salt and pepper if desired. Enjoy!

Note: You can also add additional toppings such as shredded cheese, chopped herbs, or hot sauce for extra flavor.

Quinoa Bowl with Black Beans, Roasted Vegetables, and Grilled Salmon

Ingredients:

- 1 cup quinoa
- Assorted vegetables (e.g., bell peppers, zucchini, cherry tomatoes)
- Olive oil
- Salt and pepper
- 1 can black beans, rinsed and drained
- 2 cloves garlic, minced
- 1 small onion, diced
- Vegetable broth or water
- 2 salmon fillets
- Herbs (such as parsley or dill)
- Lemon juice
- Optional toppings: avocado slices, fresh herbs, dressing

Instructions:

1. Cook the quinoa according to the package instructions and set aside.
2. Preheat the oven to a moderate temperature. Toss the assorted vegetables with olive oil, salt, and pepper. Spread them on a baking sheet and roast until they are tender and slightly caramelized.

3. While the vegetables are roasting, prepare the black beans. In a saucepan, sauté the minced garlic and diced onion in olive oil until fragrant. Add the rinsed and drained black beans along with a splash of vegetable broth or water. Simmer until the beans are heated through.
4. Season the salmon fillets with herbs, lemon juice, salt, and pepper. Grill them to your desired level of doneness.
5. Assemble the quinoa bowl by placing a generous portion of cooked quinoa at the bottom. Top it with the roasted vegetables and a scoop of the seasoned black beans.
6. Serve the quinoa bowl with a side of the grilled salmon. Optionally, you can add additional toppings such as avocado slices, fresh herbs, or a drizzle of your favorite dressing.
7. Enjoy this wholesome and flavorful Quinoa Bowl with Black Beans, Roasted Vegetables, and Grilled Salmon!

Baked Salmon with Roasted Asparagus and Quinoa

Ingredients:

- 2 salmon fillets
- Olive oil
- Salt and pepper
- 1 bunch asparagus, trimmed
- Lemon zest
- Garlic powder
- 1 cup quinoa
- Vegetable broth or water
- Fresh parsley (optional, for garnish)

Instructions:

1. Preheat the oven to a moderate temperature. Place the salmon fillets on a baking sheet lined with parchment paper. Drizzle with olive oil and season with salt and pepper.
2. Arrange the trimmed asparagus on a separate baking sheet. Drizzle with olive oil, sprinkle with lemon zest and garlic powder, and season with salt and pepper.
3. Place both baking sheets in the preheated oven and bake for about 12-15 minutes, or until the salmon is cooked through and the asparagus is tender.

4. While the salmon and asparagus are baking, cook the quinoa according to the package instructions, using vegetable broth or water for added flavor.
5. Once everything is cooked, divide the quinoa onto plates. Top with a baked salmon fillet and roasted asparagus.
6. Garnish with fresh parsley if desired. Serve and enjoy!

Apple Slices with Almond Butter

Ingredients:

- 1 large apple
- 2 tablespoons almond butter

Instructions:

1. Rinse the apple and cut it into thin slices.
2. Spread almond butter on one side of each apple slice.
3. Enjoy this simple yet nutritious snack!

Protein Shake with Banana and Peanut Butter

Ingredients:

1. 1 ripe banana
2. 2 tablespoons peanut butter
3. 1 scoop protein powder
4. 1 cup almond milk or any other milk of your choice

Instructions:

1. In a blender, combine the banana, peanut butter, protein powder, and milk.
2. Blend until smooth and creamy.
3. Pour into a glass and enjoy immediately for maximum freshness.

Roasted Chickpeas

Ingredients:

- 1 can chickpeas, rinsed and drained
- 1 tablespoon olive oil
- Salt and pepper to taste
- Optional spices: paprika, cumin, chili powder

Instructions:

1. Preheat your oven to 400°F (200°C).
2. Toss the chickpeas with olive oil, salt, pepper, and any optional spices you're using.
3. Spread the chickpeas out on a baking sheet.
4. Bake for 20-30 minutes or until crispy and golden.
5. Let them cool before enjoying it as a crunchy, protein-packed snack.

Overnight Oats with Blueberries, Almond Milk, and Protein Powder

Ingredients:

- 1/2 cup rolled oats
- 1/2 cup almond milk
- 1/2 cup fresh blueberries
- 1 scoop protein powder

Instructions:

1. In a jar or container, combine the oats, almond milk, blueberries, and protein powder.
2. Stir well to combine.
3. Cover and let sit in the fridge overnight.
4. In the morning, give it a good stir and enjoy the cold.

Green Salad with Grilled Chicken, Feta Cheese, and Light Vinaigrette

Ingredients:

- 2 cups mixed greens
- 1 grilled chicken breast, sliced
- 1/4 cup crumbled feta cheese
- Your favorite light vinaigrette

Instructions:

1. Place the mixed greens in a bowl.
2. Top with the sliced grilled chicken and crumbled feta cheese.
3. Drizzle with your favorite light vinaigrette.
4. Toss lightly to combine and serve.

Carrot Sticks with Hummus

Ingredients:

- 3 large carrots
- 1 can of chickpeas (around 15 oz.), drained and rinsed
- 2 tablespoons tahini
- 2 cloves garlic, minced
- Juice of 1 lemon
- 1/4 cup olive oil
- Salt to taste
- Optional: Paprika and fresh parsley for garnish

Instructions:

1. Thoroughly wash the carrots and cut them into stick-like pieces.
2. For the hummus, you'll start with the chickpeas. Place them in a food processor or high-powered blender.
3. Add in the tahini, minced garlic, and lemon juice.
4. While the food processor or blender is running, gradually add in the olive oil until you reach a creamy consistency. If necessary, add a little bit of water to adjust the texture.
5. Season your hummus with salt according to your preference.
6. Once done, transfer the hummus to a serving bowl. If desired, sprinkle paprika and fresh parsley on top for added color and flavor.

7. Serve your homemade hummus with the carrot sticks and enjoy this healthy and delicious snack!
8. Feel free to adjust it according to your taste or add other ingredients like roasted red peppers or cumin for a different flavor.

Baked Tilapia with Steamed Broccoli, Cauliflower, and Brown Rice

Ingredients:

- 4 tilapia fillets
- 1 head of broccoli, cut into florets
- 1 head of cauliflower, cut into florets
- 2 cups of brown rice
- Olive oil
- Salt and pepper to taste
- Lemon wedges for serving

Instructions:

1. Preheat your oven to 400°F (200°C) and line a baking tray with foil.
2. Place the tilapia fillets on the lined baking tray. Drizzle them with olive oil and season with salt and pepper. Bake for about 15-20 minutes, or until the fish is cooked through and flakes easily with a fork.
3. While the fish is baking, prepare the brown rice according to the package instructions. This usually involves combining the rice with water in a pot, bringing it to a boil, then reducing the heat and letting it simmer until the water is absorbed and the rice is tender.
4. For the vegetables, place the broccoli and cauliflower florets in a steamer basket over a pot of boiling water.

Cover and steam for about 5-7 minutes, or until the vegetables are bright green and just tender. Be careful not to overcook them – you want them to still have a bit of crunch!

5. When everything is ready, serve each tilapia fillet with a portion of steamed broccoli, cauliflower, and brown rice. Add a squeeze of fresh lemon juice over the tilapia for extra flavor, if desired.

Sample Meal Plan

With the recipes provided above, here's a sample meal plan that you can follow for a week:

Day 1: High-Calorie Day

Breakfast: Mashed sweet potato topped with sautéed spinach, mushrooms, and a fried egg.

Snack: Apple slices with almond butter.

Lunch: Quinoa bowl with black beans, roasted vegetables, and a side of grilled salmon.

Snack: Protein shake with banana and peanut butter.

Dinner: Baked salmon with roasted asparagus and a side of quinoa.

Snack: Roasted chickpeas or a small portion of dark chocolate.

Day 2: Low-Calorie Day

Breakfast: Overnight oats with blueberries, almond milk, and protein powder.

Snack: Carrot sticks with hummus.

Lunch: Green salad with grilled chicken, feta cheese, and a light vinaigrette.

Snack: Greek yogurt with fresh fruit.

Dinner: Baked tilapia with steamed broccoli, cauliflower, and a side of brown rice.

Snack: Herbal tea or a small portion of sliced melon.

Day 3: Medium-Calorie Day

Breakfast: Scrambled eggs with sautéed vegetables and a side of whole wheat toast.

Snack: Protein smoothie with banana, almond milk, and hemp seeds.

Lunch: Quinoa bowl with black beans, roasted vegetables, and a side of grilled chicken.

Snack: Apple slices with nut butter.

Dinner: Grilled salmon with roasted asparagus and a side of quinoa.

Snack: Dark chocolate squares or a small portion of mixed nuts.

Continue alternating between high, low, and medium-calorie days for the remaining four days. Remember to include a variety of nutrient-dense foods, including lean proteins, whole grains, fruits, vegetables, and healthy fats. Drink plenty of water throughout the day and listen to your body's hunger and fullness cues.

It's important to note that this is just a sample plan, and individual calorie needs may vary. It's recommended to consult with a healthcare professional or registered dietitian to create a personalized metabolic confusion diet plan that suits your specific goals and needs.

Conclusion

Congratulations! You've made it to the end of this comprehensive guide on the metabolic confusion diet for women. By reaching this point, you've taken a significant step towards understanding your body's metabolism and how you can use food as a tool to optimize its function.

Let's take a moment to recap what we've learned. The metabolic confusion diet, as we've seen, is not just another fad diet. It's a way of eating that encourages variety and flexibility, which can be a breath of fresh air in a world filled with restrictive diets. By cycling between high and low-calorie days, you keep your metabolism guessing and potentially boost its efficiency, leading to weight loss and improved health.

We've also discussed that, as a woman, your metabolic needs can vary due to factors such as hormonal changes, age, and activity level. This is why it's essential to listen to your body and adjust your diet accordingly. Remember, this is not a one-size-fits-all approach, but a guide to help you understand your body better and make informed decisions about your nutrition.

One key insight from our journey through the metabolic confusion diet is the importance of balance. While it's true that varying your caloric intake can keep your metabolism on its toes, it's equally important to ensure that you're getting a balanced mix of nutrients. This includes lean proteins, healthy fats, and a rainbow of fruits and vegetables. On both high and low-calorie days, these nutrient-dense foods should be the cornerstone of your meals.

As you embark on your metabolic confusion journey, remember that it's okay to have off days. What matters is consistency over time. Don't be discouraged if you don't see immediate results – changing your body's metabolism is a marathon, not a sprint. Celebrate small victories along the way, whether it's feeling more energetic, fitting into an old pair of jeans, or simply enjoying your meals without guilt.

Lastly, remember that while diet plays a crucial role in metabolism and weight management, it's just one piece of the puzzle. Regular exercise, adequate sleep, and stress management are equally important for maintaining a healthy metabolism and overall well-being.

In conclusion, the metabolic confusion diet offers an exciting approach to weight management and metabolic health. By providing variety and flexibility, it can be a sustainable and enjoyable way of eating that supports not just your physical health, but also your mental well-being.

So here's to you, for taking the time to learn about the metabolic confusion diet and making the commitment to better health. As you move forward, keep this guide handy as a reference,, and remember: you have the power to influence your metabolism and shape your health destiny. It's not always easy, but with perseverance and a positive attitude, it's entirely within your reach.

FAQ

What is the Metabolic Confusion diet?

The Metabolic Confusion diet is a dietary approach that involves varying your caloric intake on different days to trick your metabolism into speeding up, which may help with weight loss.

How does the Metabolic Confusion diet work?

This diet works on the principle of 'calorie cycling', where you consume more calories on some days and fewer on others. The idea is to keep your metabolism guessing, so it remains active and burns more calories.

Is the Metabolic Confusion diet safe for women?

Generally, the Metabolic Confusion diet can be safe for women, but it's crucial to ensure you're getting the right nutrients, especially on low-calorie days. However, women with certain health conditions or those who are pregnant or breastfeeding should consult their healthcare provider before starting this diet.

Can the Metabolic Confusion diet lead to nutrient deficiency?

There's a risk of nutrient deficiency, particularly on low-calorie days when you might not get enough essential nutrients. It's important to focus on nutrient-dense foods and possibly consider a multivitamin supplement under the guidance of a healthcare professional.

Can the Metabolic Confusion diet affect hormonal balance in women?

The diet, with its fluctuating caloric intake, might disrupt hormonal balance, potentially leading to issues like irregular menstrual cycles or fertility problems. Women, particularly those in their reproductive years, should consult their healthcare provider before starting this diet.

Does the Metabolic Confusion diet contribute to stress?

The constant monitoring and adjustment of caloric intake can be mentally and emotionally taxing, which could potentially heighten stress levels. If you find this diet stressful, it might not be the best approach for you.

Is the Metabolic Confusion diet a long-term solution for weight loss?

Some experts argue that the Metabolic Confusion diet might not be sustainable in the long run due to the mental and emotional strain of constantly adjusting caloric intake. For long-term weight management, a balanced, nutrient-rich diet combined with regular physical activity is often recommended.

References and Helpful Links

Gpt, S. B. N. C. C. F. (2023). What is metabolic confusion? Does it actually work? Hone Health. https://honehealth.com/edge/nutrition/metabolic-confusion-weight-loss-explained-by-dietitian/

Walter, L. (2022). Metabolic Confusion Diet Plans For Endomorphs: Full Menu. Workout Lunatic. https://workoutlunatic.com/diet/metabolic-confusion-diet-plans-for-endomorphs/

What is metabolic confusion, and is it right for you? (n.d.). https://www.joinvitalhealth.com/blog/metabolic-confusion

Metabolic syndrome - Symptoms & causes - Mayo Clinic. (2021, May 6). Mayo Clinic. https://www.mayoclinic.org/diseases-conditions/metabolic-syndrome/symptoms-causes/syc-20351916

Eikey, E. V. (2021). Effects of diet and fitness apps on eating disorder behaviours: qualitative study. British Journal of Psychiatry Open, 7(5). https://doi.org/10.1192/bjo.2021.1011

Fischer, M. (n.d.). Gainful. Gainful. https://www.gainful.com/blog/metabolic-confusion/#:~:text=For%20the%20study%20mentioned%20above,days%20of%20increased%20calorie%20consumption.

Admin. (2023, January 10). Understanding Calorie cycling | How the Metabolic Confusion diet Works in Weight Loss - Yunique Medical. Yunique Medical. https://yuniquemedical.com/calorie-cycling/

www.ingramcontent.com/pod-product-compliance
Lightning Source LLC
LaVergne TN
LVHW012035060526
838201LV00061B/4618